Erik Wissner

Utility of Intracardiac Echocardiography during Transseptal Puncture

Erik Wissner

Utility of Intracardiac Echocardiography during Transseptal Puncture

Efficacy and Outcome Analysis of Transseptal Puncture Facilitated by Phased-Array Intracardiac Echocardiography

Südwestdeutscher Verlag für Hochschulschriften

Impressum/Imprint (nur für Deutschland/ only for Germany)
Bibliografische Information der Deutschen Nationalbibliothek: Die Deutsche Nationalbibliothek verzeichnet diese Publikation in der Deutschen Nationalbibliografie; detaillierte bibliografische Daten sind im Internet über http://dnb.d-nb.de abrufbar.
 Alle in diesem Buch genannten Marken und Produktnamen unterliegen warenzeichen-, marken- oder patentrechtlichem Schutz bzw. sind Warenzeichen oder eingetragene Warenzeichen der jeweiligen Inhaber. Die Wiedergabe von Marken, Produktnamen, Gebrauchsnamen, Handelsnamen, Warenbezeichnungen u.s.w. in diesem Werk berechtigt auch ohne besondere Kennzeichnung nicht zu der Annahme, dass solche Namen im Sinne der Warenzeichen- und Markenschutzgesetzgebung als frei zu betrachten wären und daher von jedermann benutzt werden dürften.

Verlag: Südwestdeutscher Verlag für Hochschulschriften Aktiengesellschaft & Co. KG
Dudweiler Landstr. 99, 66123 Saarbrücken, Deutschland
Telefon +49 681 37 20 271-1, Telefax +49 681 37 20 271-0
Email: info@svh-verlag.de
Zugl.: Hamburg, Uni, Diss., 2009

Herstellung in Deutschland:
Schaltungsdienst Lange o.H.G., Berlin
Books on Demand GmbH, Norderstedt
Reha GmbH, Saarbrücken
Amazon Distribution GmbH, Leipzig
ISBN: 978-3-8381-1586-3

Imprint (only for USA, GB)
Bibliographic information published by the Deutsche Nationalbibliothek: The Deutsche Nationalbibliothek lists this publication in the Deutsche Nationalbibliografie; detailed bibliographic data are available in the Internet at http://dnb.d-nb.de.
 Any brand names and product names mentioned in this book are subject to trademark, brand or patent protection and are trademarks or registered trademarks of their respective holders. The use of brand names, product names, common names, trade names, product descriptions etc. even without a particular marking in this works is in no way to be construed to mean that such names may be regarded as unrestricted in respect of trademark and brand protection legislation and could thus be used by anyone.

Publisher: Südwestdeutscher Verlag für Hochschulschriften Aktiengesellschaft & Co. KG
Dudweiler Landstr. 99, 66123 Saarbrücken, Germany
Phone +49 681 37 20 271-1, Fax +49 681 37 20 271-0
Email: info@svh-verlag.de

Printed in the U.S.A.
Printed in the U.K. by (see last page)
ISBN: 978-3-8381-1586-3

Copyright © 2010 by the author and Südwestdeutscher Verlag für Hochschulschriften Aktiengesellschaft & Co. KG and licensors
All rights reserved. Saarbrücken 2010

CONTENTS

1 INTRODUCTION.. 3

    1.1 Overview... 3

    1.2 Hypothesis.. 4

    1.3 Anatomy of the Interatrial Septum............................ 4

    1.4 Historical Aspects, Development and Emerging Use of Transseptal

        Catheterization... 6

    1.5 Historical Aspects and Development of Intracardiac

        Echocardiography... 8

    1.5.1 Technical Aspects of Intracardiac Echocardiography.......... 8

    1.5.2 Protocols for Intracardiac Echocardiography Imaging........ 10

    1.5.3 Clinical Application of Intracardiac Echocardiography........ 15

    1.5.4 Intracardiac versus Transesophageal Echocardiography..... 17

2 METHODS.. 18

    2.1 Data Acquisition.. 18

    2.2 Patient Population... 19

    2.3 Procedural Aspects of Phased-Array Intracardiac

        Echocardiography.. 20

    2.4 Procedural Aspects of Transseptal Puncture............... 21

    2.5 Statistical Analysis... 22

3	RESULTS	23
	3.1 General	23
	3.2 Complications Directly Related to Transseptal Puncture	23
	3.3 Complications Not Directly Related to Transseptal Puncture	24
	3.4 Routine Next-day Transthoracic Echocardiography	25
	3.5 Influence of Left Atrial Volume Index and Enlarged Aortic Root Diameter on the Outcome of Transseptal Puncture	26
4	DISCUSSION	26
	4.1 Traditional Fluoroscopically-Guided Transseptal Puncture	27
	4.2 Adjunct Imaging Modalities to Facilitate Transseptal Puncture	28
	4.2.1 Transesophageal Echocardiography	28
	4.2.2 Intracardiac Echocardiography	28
	4.2.3 Three-Dimensional Mapping Systems	29
	4.3 Redo Transseptal Puncture	31
	4.4 Learning Curve	32
	4.5 Future Innovations	33
	4.6 Study Limitations	35
5	CONCLUSIONS	35
6	REFERENCES	37
7	ABREVIATIONS	43
8	FIGURES AND TABLES	45
9	DANKSAGUNG	48

1 INTRODUCTION

1.1 Overview

Historically, transseptal puncture (TP) was utilized by interventional cardiologists for the assessment of left atrial (LA) hemodynamics in the setting of mitral valvular disease and to allow hemodynamic assessment of the left ventricle in patients with aortic valve prostheses. Prior reports from experienced large volume centers suggested a major procedural complication rate of approximately 1.3% (1). Continued advancements in the understanding of the mechanism of atrial fibrillation (AF), along with a persistent evolution of ablation approaches for treatment of this arrhythmia, has led to an ever growing need for LA access. In fact, the ubiquitous nature of AF in addition to the acknowledgement that the vast majority of curative endocardial ablation approaches for the treatment of AF are now performed within the LA, have virtually ensured that the TP procedure will remain an integral part of the procedural armamentarium of the interventional cardiac electrophysiologist for the unforeseen future. The current practice at many centers is to still utilize fluoroscopy as the sole form of imaging employed for visualization during performance of TP (2-5). It is clear that there are distinct inherent limitations regarding the accuracy of intracardiac catheter placement and manipulation when utilizing only fluoroscopic visualization. These potential inaccuracies may be further amplified in patients with significant structural heart disease or derangements of chamber dimensions. Use of intracardiac echocardiography (ICE) imaging to facilitate TP not only aids in a potentially more accurate placement of the transseptal sheath within the LA, but also provides incrementally greater and possibly more accurate imaging data regarding the interatrial septum/fossa ovalis, surrounding adjacent cardiac structures, and a more immediate ability to assess for complications (6).

1.2 Hypothesis

Due to a paucity of data in larger cohorts of patients regarding the impact of ICE imaging during TP, this study sought to assess the feasibility and influence of phased-array ICE guidance on the outcome of TP during ablation procedures in the electrophysiology (EP) laboratory.

1.3 Anatomy of the Interatrial Septum

A thorough understanding of the cardiac anatomy is needed to perform safe TP. The interatrial septum is formed by the remnants of septum primum and secundum, extending from superior to inferior towards the endocardial cushion. The septum primum is absorbed superiorly so that the septum secundum forms this part of the interatrial septum. Fusion of both septi results in formation of the limbus, the raised margin of the fossa ovalis. The fossa ovalis measures on average 1.5 to 2.4 cm^2 and consists of thin fibrous tissue (7) . The foramen ovale allows right to left blood flow in the fetal circulation. After birth functional closure takes place caused by increasing left atrial pressures. Anatomic closure follows; however, in up to 25% of the general population the foramen ovale remains patent. This may become clinically significant if right-sided intracardiac pressures supersede left atrial pressure, allowing shunting of blood from right to left surpassing the pulmonary circulation thus facilitating the occurrence of paradoxical embolism. **See Figure 1.**

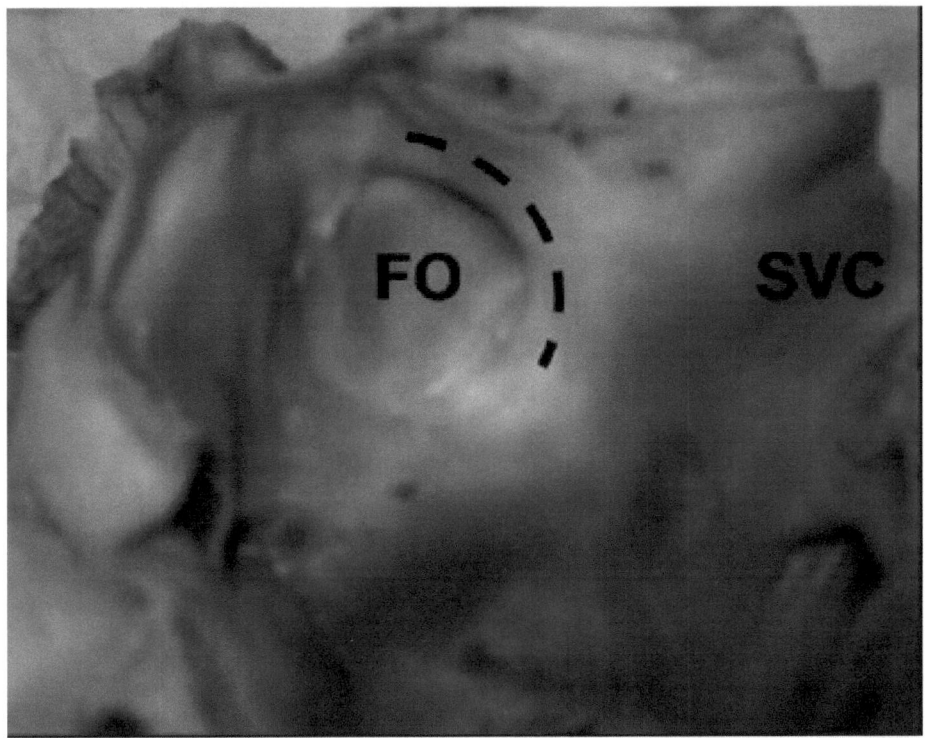

Figure 1. Interatrial septum and limbus encircling the fossa ovalis seen from a right atrial view (from (8))

1.4 Historical Aspects, Development and Emerging Use of Transseptal Catheterization

The era of transseptal catheterization began in 1957 when Dr. Ross, at the time resident in surgery at John's Hopkins Hospital and temporarily working at the National Institute of Health under the auspices of Dr. Morrow, carried out experiments in dogs to measure left atrial and ventricular pressures. He used a long curved needle inserted through the dog's saphenous vein to access the left atrium via the interatrial septum. These animal experiments followed the first clinical application in man published in 1959 (9). Dr. Brockenbrough, also working at the National Institute of Health, modified the transseptal needle to allow insertion via the Seldinger technique and published his data in 1960 and 1962 (10,11) (see **Figure 2**). Other clinical studies followed. Transseptal catheterization became routine during mitral valve balloon valvuloplasty and presently is part of the armamentarium of the interventional electrophysiologist involved in procedures necessitating mapping and ablation within the left sided heart chambers.

Emerging indications for TP include percutaneous repair of atrial septal defects or closure of a patent foramen ovale in patients with proven right to left shunting resulting in paradoxical embolism. Other indications are percutaneous mitral valve repair and percutaneous closure of paravalvular leaks of mitral valves prostheses. Left atrial appendage closure devices for the prevention of stroke are placed via a TP approach. Finally, TP is necessary for the treatment of pulmonary vein stenosis following atrial fibrillation ablation procedures, in order to allow for balloon angioplasty and/or stent placement.

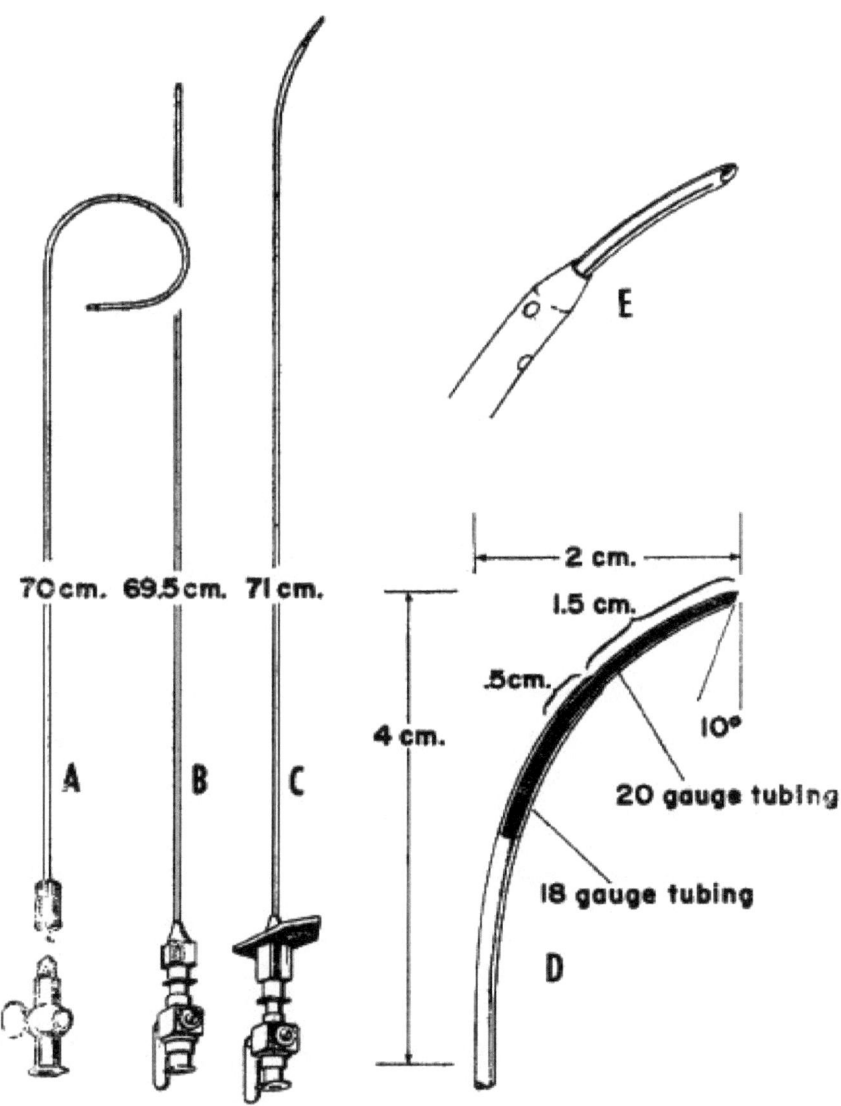

Figure 2. Original setup used in Dr. Brockenbrough's study describing transseptal catheterization in 450 patients. Needle 'C' shows the Brockenbrough needle used today.

1.5 Historical Aspects and Development of Intracardiac Echocardiography

Fluoroscopy is the primary visualization tool in the EP laboratory allowing for 2-dimensional imaging of cardiac structures. However, fluoroscopy does not provide visualization of cardiac soft tissue while radiation exposure poses health risks to patients and health care professionals. These disadvantages led to the development of alternative imaging modalities. Intracardiac echocardiography first developed and applied in humans in 1994 is now routinely utilized in 50% of centers performing atrial fibrillation ablation procedures (12,13).

1.5.1 Technical Aspects of Intracardiac Echocardiography

Two types of ICE transducers are currently commercially available. The mechanical (rotational) ICE transducer is offered as a 6-9 Fr catheter with a single ultrasound crystal mounted at the distal tip of a nonsteerable catheter (12,14). A drive unit rotates the crystal within the catheter allowing for a circumferential and perpendicular imaging field with a depth of up to 7 cm (15). The poor remote tissue penetration is due to the high imaging frequency (9 to 12 MHz) utilized. Phased-array ICE catheters are available in either 8 or 10 Fr (16). The four-way head articulation allows multiple angle imaging, giving a 90° wedge shaped imaging field with tissue penetration as deep as 10-12 cm (17). In addition to two-dimensional imaging, phased-array ICE offers M-mode, pulsed, continuous and color Doppler capabilities. **Table 1** provides an overview of the different characteristics of the available ICE transducers.

Table 1. Comparison between Mechanical (Rotational) and Phased-Array ICE (adapted from (15,18))

Characteristic	Mechanical (Rotational)	Phased-Array
Plane of View	Horizontal only	90° angle
Depth of Imaging Field	Maximum of 7 cm	Adjustable between 2 - 12 cm
Doppler Capabilities	No	Color, Continuous and Pulse Wave
Deflectable Catheter Tip	No	Yes
Available Size	6-9 French	8 or 10 French

ICE, Intracardiac Echocardiography

1.5.2 Protocols for Phased-Array ICE Imaging

General approach

The femoral vein is typically utilized for the insertion of the ICE catheter with the operator standing at the patient's right side.

"Home" view

After advancing the catheter carefully from the inferior vena cava to the mid-right atrium, the transducer is rotated gently anteriorly to provide the "home" view. In this view the right atrium, right ventricle and tricupid valve are displayed. See **Figure 3**.

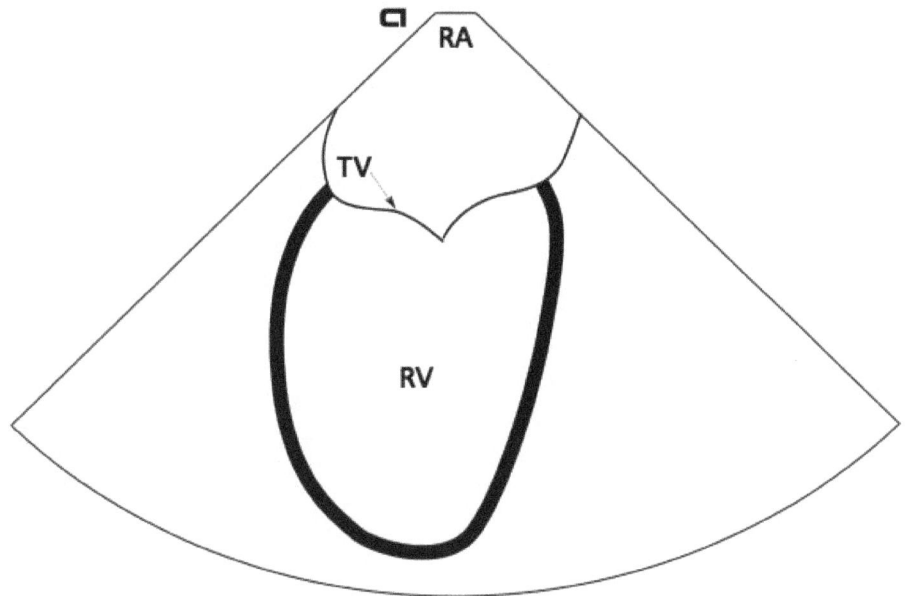

Figure 3. The "home" view displays right atrium, right ventricle and tricuspid valve. *RA*, right atrium; *TV*, tricuspid valve; *RV*, right ventricle.

Intra-atrial septum and fossa ovalis

The catheter is rotated clockwise, away from the operator and slightly advanced or tilted posteriorly as needed (**Figure 4**).

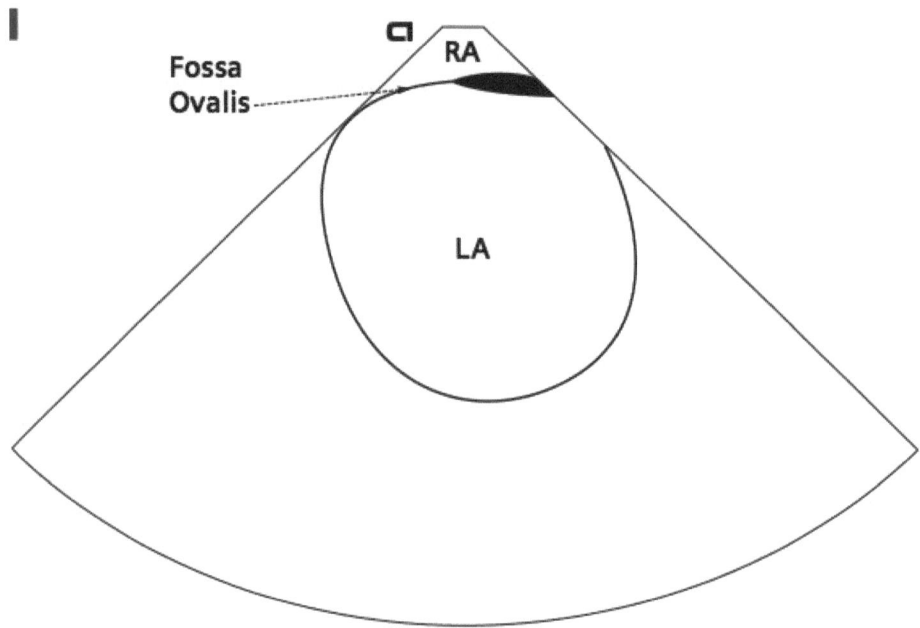

Figure 4. View of intra-atrial septum and fossa ovalis. *RA*, right atrium; *LA*, left atrium.

Left pulmonary veins

From the intra-atrial septum/fossa ovalis view, the operator advances the ICE catheter superiorly in order to visualize the left pulmonary veins (**Figure 5**).

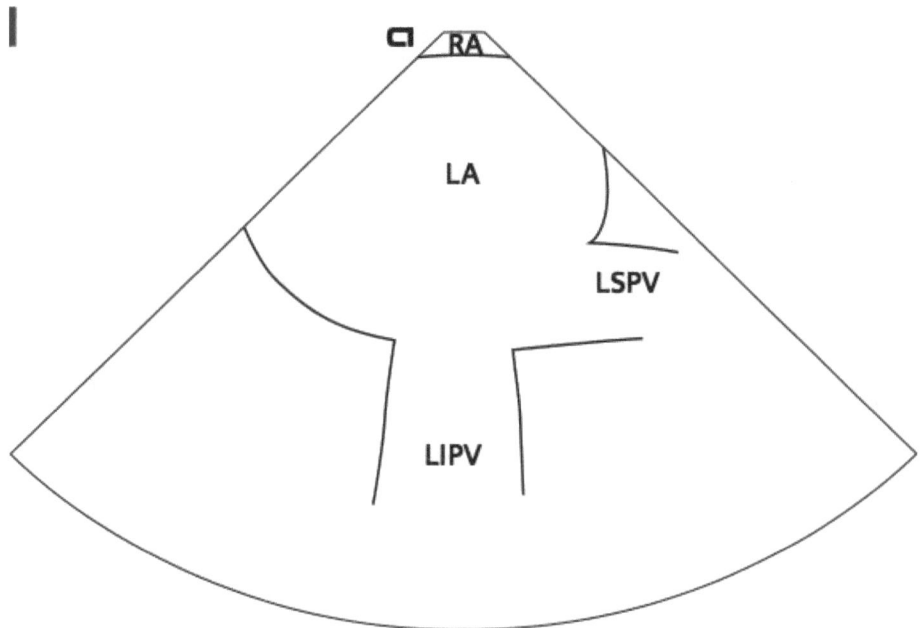

Figure 5. View of superior and inferior left pulmonary veins. *RA*, right atrium; *LA*, left atrium; *LSPV*, left superior pulmonary vein; *LIPV*, left inferior pulmonary vein.

Right pulmonary veins

Rotating and advancing the catheter clockwise past the left pulmonary veins will display the right pulmonary veins (**Figure 6**).

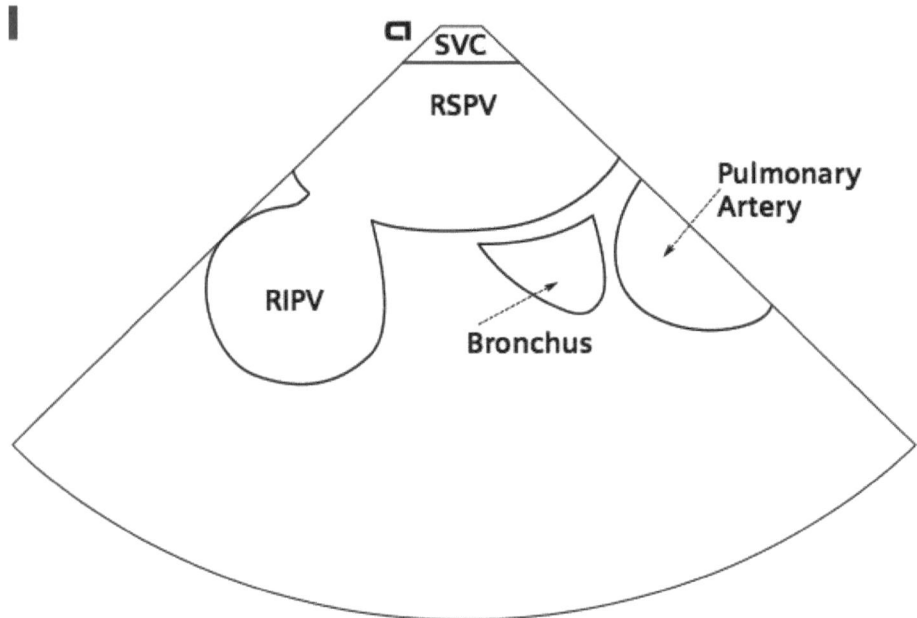

Figure 6. View of right superior and inferior pulmonary veins. *SVC*, superior vena cava; *RSPV*, right superior pulmonary vein; *RIPV*, right inferior pulmonary vein.

Assessment of pericardial effusion

In order to assess for pericardial effusion, the operator withdraws the catheter to the inferior right atrium and then advances anteriorly past the tricuspid valve into the right ventricle (**Figure 7**).

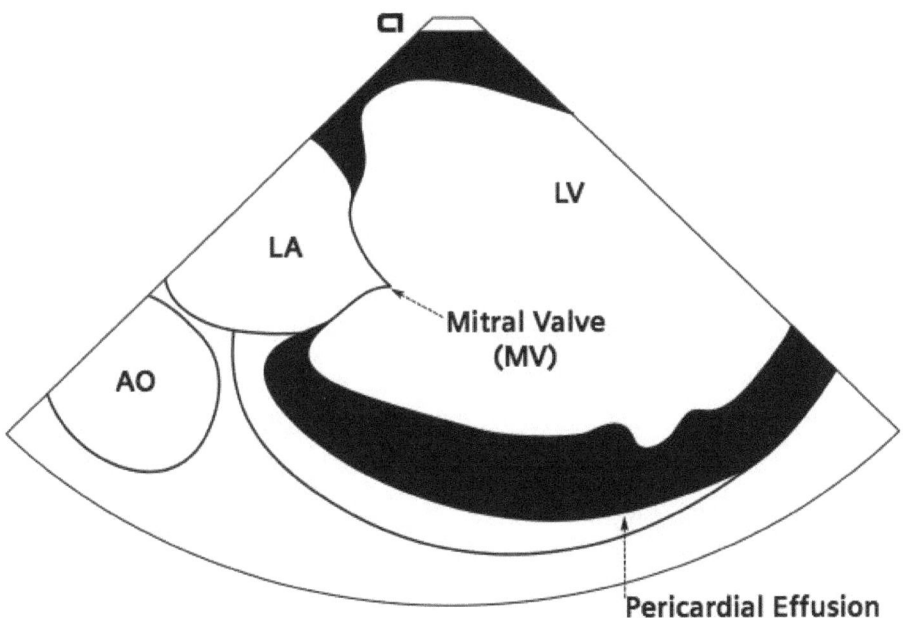

Figure 7. Left ventricle in long axis view for the assessment of pericardial effusion. *LV*, left ventricle; *LA*, left atrium; *AO*, aorta; *MV*, mitral valve.

1.5.3 Clinical Application of Intracardiac Echocardiography

Since ICE accurately defines soft tissue structures, the operator is provided with a tool that readily identifies the mapping/ablation catheter within the heart. This in turn facilitates catheter navigation, verification of catheter-tissue contact and lesion formation (19,20). In addition, ICE directly visualizes ablation catheter placement along the PV and helps identifying the PV ostia to allow exact placement of the circular multipolar PV mapping catheter at the LA/PV ostial border. ICE serves as a screening tool for bubble formation during ablation (21). Bubble formation has shown to be a surrogate marker of tissue overheating (22).

Furthermore, ICE allows visualization of the transseptal needle within the right atrium prior puncture of the fossa ovalis, thus assuring accurate alignment of needle and sheath. Consequently, the exact position of puncture, e.g. anterior or posterior along the fossa ovalis may be selected. This in turn may facilitate maneuverability of sheath and catheter. Variants of atrial septal anatomy such as septal aneurysm or lipomatous hypertrophy can readily be identified (**Figure 8**).

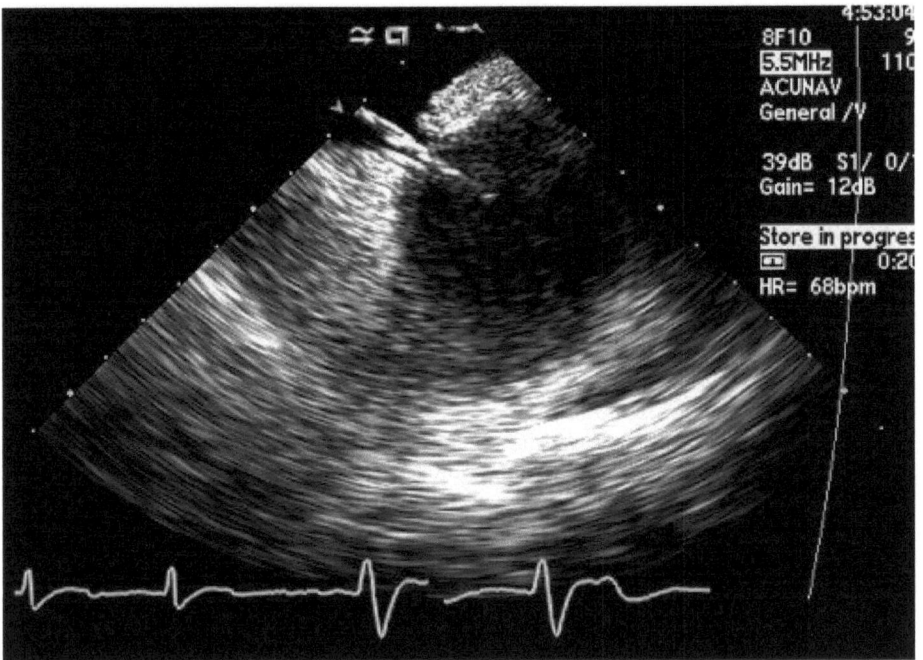

Figure 8. Intracardiac echocardiography image demonstrating a lipomatous septum with transseptal catheter traversing a narrow fossa ovalis

Measurements of intracardiac structures such as length of right atrial cavotricuspid isthmus (23) or pulmonary vein ostial diameter before and after PV isolation are promptly available. ICE accurately identifies all existing PV ostia and their diameters when compared to cardiac computed tomography (24). Since phased-array ICE offers Doppler capabilities, PV flow velocities may be assessed, providing the operator with valuable information regarding the potential for PV stenosis (25).

The existence and development of intraoperative intracardiac thrombus is easily detectable with ICE (26). It may also facilitate the identification of abnormal structures, which technically limit ablation within the left atrium (19).

ICE imaging allows delineation of the course of the esophagus and its distance to the left atrium. Structures within the right atrium not readily seen on fluoroscopy such as the crista terminalis can be visualized using ICE and thus facilitate ablation of atrial tachycardias arising from this structure (27).

Intraprocedural complications such as development of a pericardial effusion or tamponade are immediately assessable using ICE. Finally, in patients with congenital heart disease surgical baffles or patches serving as arrhythmogenic material may be visualized with ICE. See **Table 2**.

Table 2. Clinical Application of Intracardiac Echocardiography

---

- Catheter navigation
- Visualization during transseptal puncture
- Identification of cardiac anatomy
- Visualization of pulmonary vein ostia
- Identification of electrode-tissue contact
- Assessment of flow velocities by pulse/continuous wave and color flow Doppler
- Assessment of bubble formation and lesion formation
- Visualization of esophageal-left atrial continuity
- Identification of potential complications
    - Thrombus formation
    - Pericardial effusion
    - Tissue overheating
    - Pulmonary vein stenosis

1.5.4 Intracardiac versus Transesophageal Echocardiography

Although transesophageal echocardiography is readily available at most medical centers, it bears several disadvantages. Intracardiac echocardiography offers superior imaging quality and may result in an overall safer procedure. Additionally, sedation is needed during prolonged procedures utilizing TEE but is not required during ICE-guided procedures. However, the ICE catheter is intended for single use only, while TEE transducers can be reutilized following proper sterilization. Cardiac imaging utilizing TEE necessitates the expertise of a second operator familiar with the intricacies of echocardiography. In contrast, a single operator may perform ICE evaluation in addition to mapping and ablation.

2 METHODS

2.1 Data Acquisition

A retrospective review of each consecutive patient's medical record was employed, analyzing baseline pre-procedural characteristics, EP study reports, occurrence of procedural complications, and pre- and postprocedural transthoracic echocardiography data. A complete EP study data set (including details regarding the TP and ICE) was available for all patients, while transthoracic echocardiography data varied according to the type of ablation procedure performed (typically only patients undergoing AF ablation would undergo routine next-day limited echocardiographic evaluation to assess for pericardial effusion, unless otherwise specified). Patients without an EP indication for TP or LA access obtained via a patent foramen ovale were excluded from the study protocol. Each TP was performed by one of three board certified invasive cardiac electrophysiologists or alternatively by one cardiac electrophysiology fellow in training under staff physician supervision. The Mayo Clinic Arizona institutional review board approved this analysis and the need for informed consent was waived.

2.2 Patient Population

The study cohort consisted of 167 consecutive patients (mean age 60 ± 11 years; 36% female; body mass index [BMI] 29 ± 6) referred for EP study with mapping and ablation requiring access to the LA or left ventricle between February 2004 and April 2008. TP was performed to facilitate ablation for atrial fibrillation in 82.6% of patients, atrioventricular reentrant tachycardia in 5.4%, atrial tachycardia in 4.8%, atypical atrial flutter in 3.6%, atypical atrioventricular nodal reentrant tachycardia in 2.4%, and ventricular tachycardia or premature ventricular contractions in 1.2% of patients. Baseline characteristics and echocardiographic data are summarized in **Table 3**. The type of procedure and number of patients with redo procedures are listed in **Table 4** and **Table 5**, respectively.

Table 3. Patients' Baseline Demographic & Echocardiographic Data, N=167 (%)	
Age (years)	60 ± 11
Female gender	60 (36)
Body Mass Index	29 ± 6
Hypertension	85 (51)
Ischemic Cardiomyopathy	3 (2)
Nonischemic Cardiomyopathy	7 (4)
Permanent Pacemaker or Implantable Cardioverter Defibrillator in Situ	15 (9)
LVEF (%)	61 ± 9
LAVI (cc/m^2)	33 ± 10
Aortic root diameter (mm)	34 ± 5

LVEF, Left Ventricular Ejection Fraction; *LAVI*, Left Atrial Volume Index

Table 4. Type of Procedure Among the Cohort of Patients (N=167)		
Atrial Fibrillation Ablation	138	82.6%
Atrial Tachycardia Ablation	8	4.8%
Orthodromic AVRT Ablation	7	4.2%
Atypical Atrial Flutter Ablation	6	3.6%
Atypical AVNRT Ablation	4	2.4%
WPW Ablation	2	1.2%
VT Ablation	1	0.6%
PVC Ablation	1	0.6%

AVRT, Atrioventricular Reentry Tachycardia; *AVNRT*, Atrioventricular Nodal Reentry Tachycardia; *WPW*, Wolff-Parkinson-White; *VT*, Ventricular Tachycardia; *PVC*, Premature Ventricular Contraction

Table 5. Number of Patients with Redo Procedures		
None	142	85%
1 Redo Procedure	23	13.8%
2 Redo Procedures	2	1.2%

2.3 Procedural Aspects of Phased-Array Intracardiac Echocardiography

An 8 or 10 French phased-array ICE catheter (AcuNav, Acuson, Mountain View, CA, USA) was introduced via a femoral venous approach in all patients. The ICE catheter was advanced to the right atrium and stably situated. The catheter was set in a neutral position using a depth of 110 cm to allow visualization of the interatrial septum. This position usually permits a thorough delineation and visualization of the interatrial septum. Using this setting, true engagement of the fossa ovalis (excluding the muscular interatrial septum) could be more accurately certified, as well as micro-bubble or clot formation, and final sheath location within the LA. Finally, immediate complications related to TP, such as inadvertent cannulation of nearby structures (aorta, pericardial space, etc) or development of pericardial effusion could readily be visualized.

2.4 Procedural Aspects of Transseptal Puncture

The right femoral vein was cannulated using the modified Seldinger technique and a 135 cm, 0.0352" (0.813 mm) guidewire (St. Jude Medical, Minnetonka, MN, USA)) was advanced to the superior vena cava. A 63 cm long 8 French sheath (SL0 or SL1, St. Jude Medical, Minnetonka, MN, USA) with dilator was advanced over the guidewire to the superior vena cava. This step was typically repeated for the second transseptal sheath. Following removal of the guidewire, a 71 cm transseptal needle (Brk-1, St. Jude Medical, Minnetonka, MN, USA) was advanced into the first transseptal sheath to within 1.0 cm proximal to the tip of the dilator sheath. Using left and right anterior oblique fluoroscopic views and ICE guidance, the TP needle and sheath (oriented in a 3 to 6 o'clock position) were gradually withdrawn as one unit until the foramen ovale was successfully engaged. Following this the TP needle was advanced out of the dilator sheath using fluoroscopic and ICE visualization. ICE imaging confirmed micro-bubbles within the LA, which were demonstrated when flushing the TP needle immediately following LA access. Finally, a LA pressure waveform and measurement were used for verification.

The dilator was then advanced over the needle into the mid-LA, with the needle fixed, and then the guide sheath was advanced over the dilator and positioned stably within the LA **(Figure 8)**. After removal of needle and dilator, an ablation/mapping catheter was placed through the sheath and into the LA. As noted above, in most patients undergoing AF ablation therapy a second TP was performed utilizing a second sheath in the same fashion. Weight based heparin therapy was then administered utilizing a bolus followed by a continuous infusion, targeting an activated clotting time of 300-350 seconds.

2.5 Statistical Analysis

Continuous variables are presented as means ± standard deviation. Since the distribution of the continuous data (tested with Kolmogorov-Smirnov Z) did not resemble normal distribution, the nonparametric Mann-Whitney U-test was used for comparison of continuous variables. Categorical variables were compared using Chi-square test. Data were analyzed using SPSS 15.0 for Windows. A P value of < 0.05 was considered statistically significant.

3 RESULTS

3.1 General

A total of 308 TPs were performed in 167 patients (123 patients underwent double TP). Twenty-five of the patients underwent 27 repeat procedures (21 of the 27 repeat procedures involved double TP) **(Table 6)**.

Table 6. Transseptal Punctures

	Patients	# TP	# Procedures	# TP-Related Complications
All	167	308 (123D, 62S)	185	1
First TP	158	260 (102D, 56S)	158	1
Redo TP	25	48 (21D, 6S)	27	0

TP, Transseptal puncture; *D*, Double; *S*, Single; #, Number

3.2 Complications Directly Related to Transseptal Puncture

A single complication (rate of 0.3% per TP; 0.6% per patient) occurred in 308 TPs performed. This patient suffered a probable perforation of the lateral LA wall induced by the TP sheath, which resulted in the acute development of a hemodynamically unstable pericardial effusion. The patient was successfully treated with acute reversal of anticoagulation and pericardiocentesis. The procedure was abandoned, requiring no surgical intervention and an uncomplicated AF ablation was performed at a future date.

3.3 Complications Not Directly Related to Transseptal Puncture

No complications were noted in the 25 patients referred for repeat procedures, nor were any noted among the 63 (20.5%) TPs performed in 38

(32.4%) patients by the electrophysiology fellow under direct staff physician supervision. There were three complications, which occurred in 3 (1.8%) patients during AF ablation therapy. As these complications occurred remotely after the TP, it is assumed that neither occurrence was directly related to the TP. The first patient suffered a perforation at the junction of right atrium and ventricle at the level of the coronary sinus during performance of a cavotricuspid isthmus lesion set, which required surgical intervention. The second patient developed a small pericardial effusion within 1 hour after completion of the AF ablation procedure, which was treated conservatively. Finally, the third patient suffered cardiac tamponade within 1 hour after completion of the AF ablation procedure. Surgical intervention was required demonstrating a laceration of the lateral left atrium in the region of a mitral isthmus lesion set. See **Table 7**.

Table 7. Intraprocedural Complications Among the Patient Cohort (N=167)

None	154	97.6%
Cardiac Perforation with Tamponade	2	1.2%
Cardiac perforation	1	0.6%
Pericardial Effusion	1	0.6%

3.4 Routine Next-Day Transthoracic Echocardiography

Of the 118 (70.7%) patients who underwent limited, routine next-day transthoracic echocardiographic evaluation, 10 (8 small, 1 moderate and 1 large) pericardial effusions not seen intraoperatively were demonstrable. Only the large pericardial effusion required pericardiocentesis. No surgical intervention was necessary in any of these situations. See **Table 8** and **9**.

Table 8. Pericardial Effusions Noted During Next Day Limited Echocardiographic Evaluation in 118 Patients	
No Effusion	65
Trivial	43
Small	8
Moderate	1
Large	1

Table 9. Pericardial Effusions Noted During Next Day Limited Echocardiographic Evaluation in 20 Redo Patients	
No Effusion	15
Trivial	3
Small	2
Moderate	0
Large	0

3.5 Influence of Left Atrial Volume Index and Enlarged Aortic Root Diameter on the Outcome of Transseptal Puncture

Table 10 depicts echocardiographic parameters analyzed for significant impact on the outcome of TP. Neither increased LA volume (LA volume index > 28 cc/m^2), underlying cardiomyopathy, increased BMI, nor an enlarged aortic root diameter (> 39 mm) correlated with an increased complication rate during TP.

Table 10. Echocardiographic Parameters

	Minimum	Maximum	Mean	Standard Deviation
LA Volume Index (cc/m^2)	14	78	33	10
LVEF (%)	22	82	61	9
Aortic Root Diameter (mm)	23	60	34	5

LA, Left atrial; LVEF, Left ventricular ejection fraction

4 DISCUSSION

This study demonstrates that ICE facilitated TP is feasible providing a wealth of additional information such as visualization of potential intraprocedural complications. The herein reported complication rate of 0.6% per patient or 0.3% per TP is in line with historical data. Furthermore, safe TP is possible even in patients with variant anatomy such as a lipomatous hypertrophy of the interatrial septum.

4.1 Traditional Fluoroscopically Guided Transseptal Puncture

Currently fluoroscopy continues to serve as the sole means of image guidance during TP at many medical centers (2-5). A large single center retrospective review of 1279 patients undergoing fluoroscopically guided TP reported a complication rate of 1.36% with cardiac tamponade representing the majority of adverse events (1). Another large retrospective analysis from Italy involving 1150 patients found no acute complications related to TP, although 2.7% of patients demonstrated trivial/small to moderate pericardial effusions (4). Of these patients, pericardial tamponade requiring pericardiocentesis was noted in 1% of the patients at the end of the procedure. As no transesophageal or intracardiac echocardiographic imaging was used at the time of TP, it is unclear whether these complications were related to TP itself or related to their subsequent AF ablation procedures. In a third study, De Ponti et al. assessed the safety of a simplified approach to TP utilizing radiographic guidance (28). Among 411 patients, 2 patients experienced inappropriate puncture of the right atrial free wall without associate untoward consequences. The same author reported on a multicenter survey conducted in Italy spanning 12 years, noting a procedural complication rate of 0.76%, which included one mortality related to the procedure (3). Centers in this particular study used a variety of imaging techniques including fluoroscopy, ICE (the particular technology utilized was not clearly specified) and transesophageal echocardiography; however details of fluoroscopy only versus ICE facilitated TP related complications were not provided. To date, no prospective study has assessed the feasibility and safety of TP using the traditional fluoroscopic approach. Additionally, no head-to-head comparison has been performed comparing different imaging modalities to facilitate TP. The current study of 167 patients reporting a complication rate of 0.6% is in line with studies utilizing merely fluoroscopic guidance for TP.

4.2 Adjunct Imaging Modalities Utilized During Transseptal Puncture

4.2.1 Transesophageal Echocardiography

Transesophageal echocardiography (TEE) guided TP offers the additional benefit of intraprocedural thrombus detection (29,30) However, the need for esophageal intubation exposes the patient to the additional risk of esophageal perforation and the lack of direct manipulation by the primary operator limits the role of TEE as an adjunct to transseptal catheterization.

4.2.2 Intracardiac Echocardiography

The advent of phased-array ICE has provided the interventional electrophysiologist with a tool that is effortlessly used by a single operator and provides immediate visualization of surrounding structures as well as immediate assessment for possible complications (6). Three studies to date have reported no complications in patients undergoing ICE facilitated TP (31-33). Although these studies report no complications, they are limited by small numbers of patients, as exemplified by the fact that the current study enrolled more patients than all previous studies combined (167 versus 115 patients).

In contrast to these studies, the current study included patients undergoing redo ablation procedures, involved procedures performed by a fellow in training, and involved patients with structural heart disease.

This study finds that the use of ICE allows for more optimal placement of single or double transseptal sheaths within the LA. This may potentially lead to greater ease of catheter manipulation, as well as more accurate, anatomically defined positioning within the LA. In addition, ICE allows assessment of nearby structures during and after TP. In patients with normal LA size, inadvertent puncture of the LA wall may be prevented by direct echocardiographic visualization. In the current study, LA size did not correlate with an increased complication rate. Furthermore, aortic root enlargement may increase the risk of aortic puncture and lead to abandonment of the planned atrial fibrillation procedure (34). Although 13 (7.8%) patients in the current study had known aortic root enlargement measuring greater than 39 mm, this finding did not translate into an increased complication rate during ICE facilitated TP.

4.2.3 Three-Dimensional Mapping Systems

Data is lacking in larger patient cohorts on alternative imaging modalities facilitating TP. An unconventional method to TP using the 3-dimensional mapping system NavX (St. Jude Medical) was reported in a case report by Shepherd et al (35). The authors used a conventional Brockenbrough needle inserted via a sheath and dilator in combination with the NavX system. In order to visualize the tip of the TP needle the distal upper half of the plastic cover of the dilator was removed, allowing registration of the needle tip along the interatrial septum after completion of a right atrial 3-dimensional map (see **Figure 9**). TP was completed without complications.

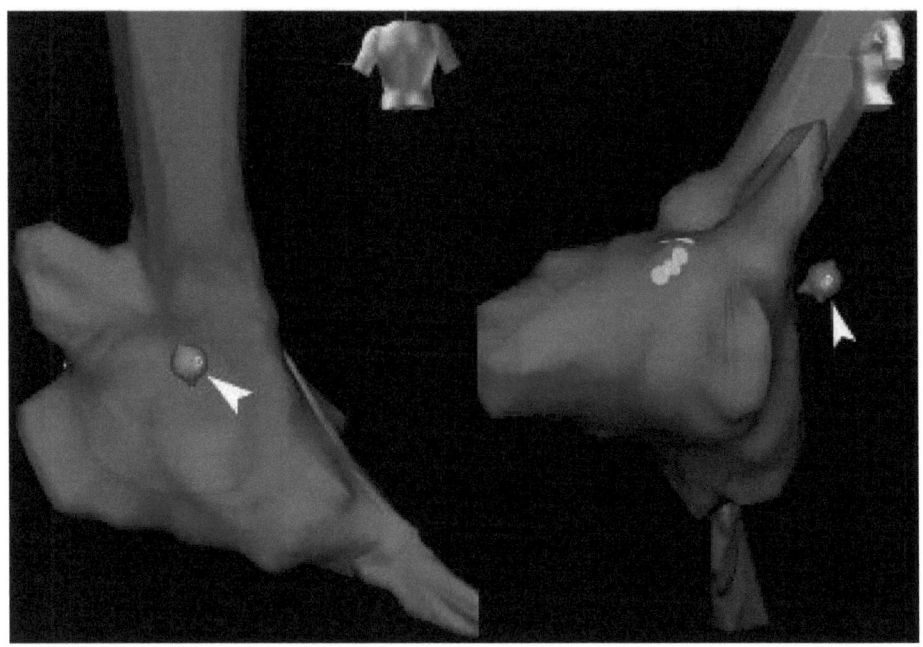

Figure 9. Right atrial NavX map with tenting of the needle tip visualized along the fossa ovalis (white arrow head; yellow dots mark the His bundle position). From (35)

The feasibility of integrating electroanatomic mapping and ICE (CartoSound, Biosense Webster) was recently demonstrated (36). Incorporating an electroanatomic sensor within the tip of the phased-array intracardiac ultrasound catheter allows creation of 3-dimensional volumes and real-time visualization of catheters and sheaths. Compared to preregistered cardiac CT images used for electroanatomic image integration (e.g. CartoMerge, Biosense Webster), this method provides real-time volume rendering obtained from within the right atrium.

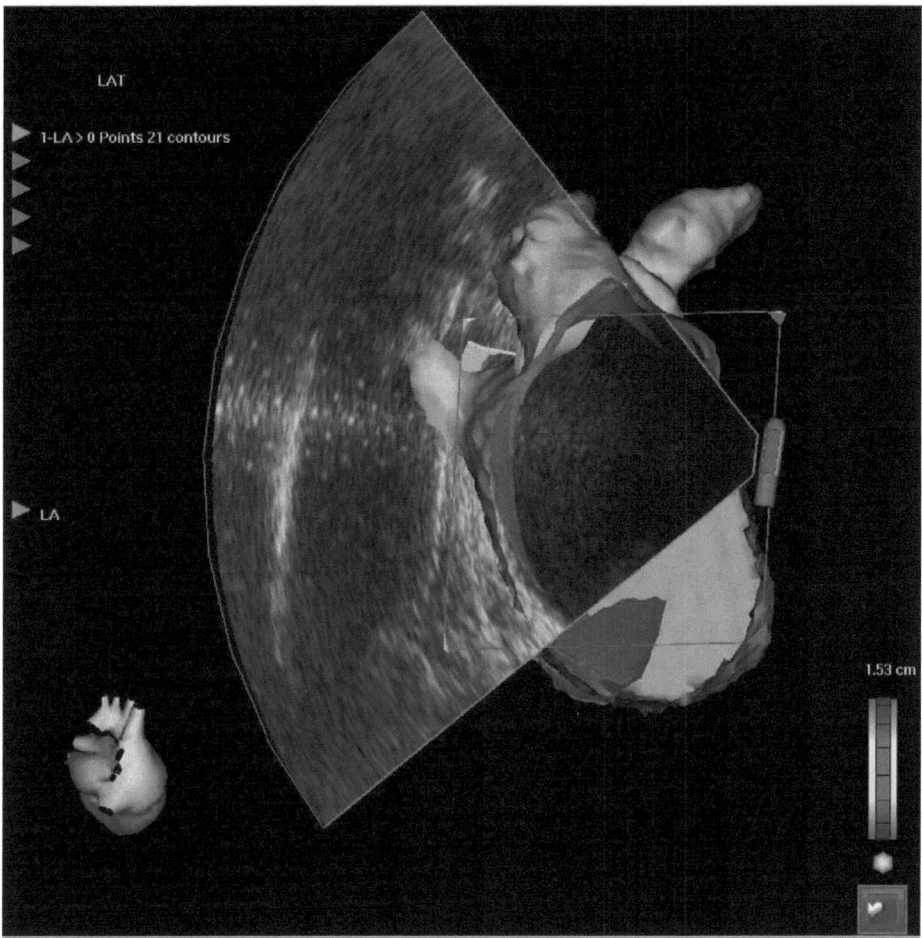

Figure 10. CartoSound (Biosense Webster) image of the left atrium realized through integration of ICE imaging and electroanatomic mapping. In addition, CT image integration visualizing the pulmonary veins is shown. From (37)

4.3 Redo Transseptal Puncture

A recent study showed that repeat, traditional TP in 29 patients during a second atrial fibrillation procedure was more difficult, necessitating the use of a large-curve transseptal needle (38). Additionally, Marcus et al. reported on 16 patients undergoing repeat TP utilizing ICE imaging (39). In 5 out of their 16 patients, repeat TP was more difficult and in 3 patients ultimately unsuccessful. In this series, one inadvertent posterior atrial puncture occurred. In contrast, the current study reports no complications during 48 redo TPs in 25 patients. Although difficult TPs in this patient subgroup were not specifically analyzed, TP may be more challenging and more commonly necessitate repositioning of the TP needle along the fossa ovalis during these procedures.

4.4 Learning Curve

Among various studies assessing the role of ICE in the EP laboratory, only few analyzed the learning curve involved in successful use of ICE during transseptal catheterization (6,33). Johnson et al. demonstrated a statistically significant correlation between operator experience and fewer attempts to successful TP facilitated by phased-array ICE in dogs (6). Additionally, Villacastin et al. concluded in their study, comprising 50 patients, that ICE facilitated the learning process mainly due to direct visualization of anatomic structures (33). According to the author's experience, ICE enhances the understanding and conceptualization of intricate cardiac anatomy and eases the steep learning curve for the inexperienced physician. This is underscored by the fact that the participation of an electrophysiology fellow in nearly 25% of all TPs did not result in a single TP related complication.

4.5 Future Innovations

With the advent of 3-dimensional echocardiography, intracardiac structures can be displayed in real-time, giving a new dimension to intraoperative imaging. Three-dimensional transesophageal echocardiography allows direct visualization of transseptal puncture and subsequent placement of mapping and ablation catheter within the left atrium (40). See **Figure 11A and 11B**. Due to the complexities of 3-dimensional imaging, ICE imaging still awaits integration of this new technique.

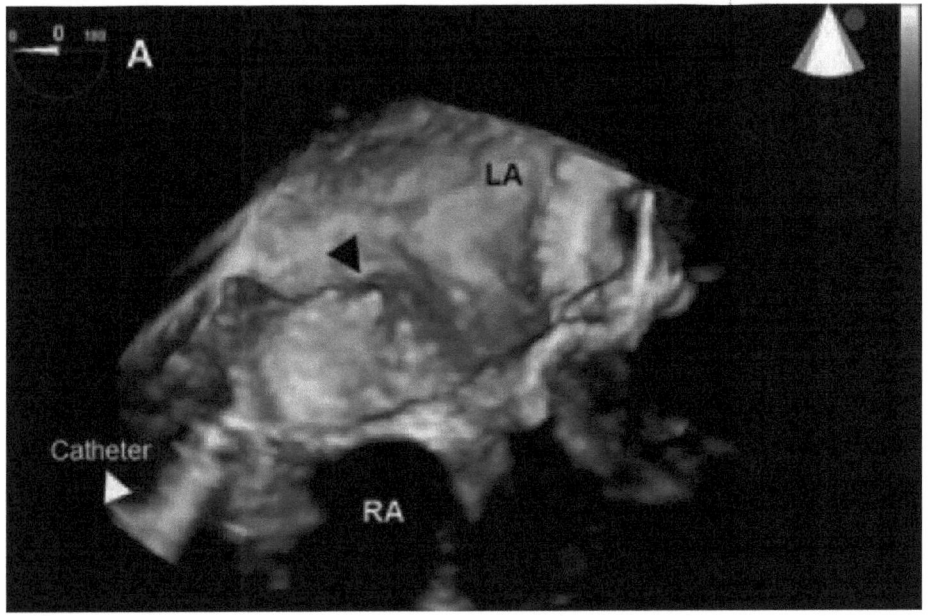

Figure 11A. Tenting of the fossa ovalis (black arrow head) by the transseptal catheter tip (white arrow head) as seen from the left atrial perspective. From (40)

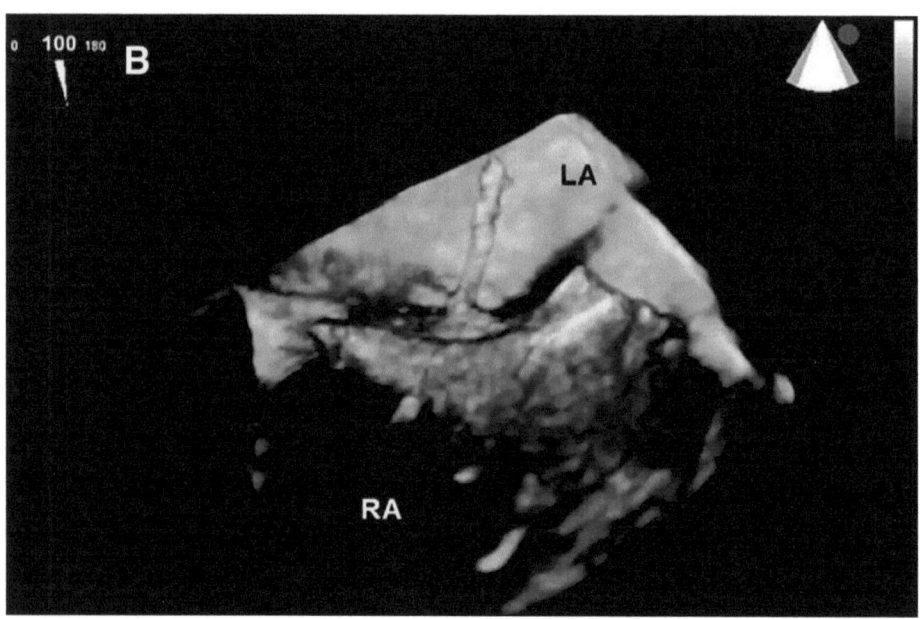

Figure 11B. The ablation catheter is visualized traversing the intra-atrial septum from right to left atrium following successful transseptal puncture. From (40)

Direct visualization of the fossa ovalis through use of a fiberoptic catheter (CardioOptics, Inc. Mass, USA) that emits infrared light allowing direct visualization of cardiac structures through blood may facilitate difficult transseptal punctures in the future.

Bidart et al. described a novel concept performing TP using an electrocautery device commonly used during surgical procedures. Radiofrequency energy using the "cutting" mode was applied to the proximal shaft of the TP needle with successful penetration of the fossa ovalis in all patients (41). Knecht et al. described a similar technique using the ablation catheter as power source for RF energy delivery to the proximal shaft of the

TP needle (42) The particular advantage of this technique may apply to patients referred for redo atrial fibrillation ablation procedures, when easy transseptal access is hampered by a fibrotic septum.

4.6 Study Limitations

The current study is a retrospective analysis with its inherent limitations. A prospective study is needed to fully evaluate and compare the complication rate of traditional fluoroscopically guided TP and ICE facilitated TP. Fluoroscopy was utilized to position the ICE catheter and the TP sheath. This study did not analyze the number of attempts to successful ICE facilitated TP. The inexperienced operator may require several attempts to properly position the TP sheath along the fossa ovalis. This may add to the procedure duration, a factor that was not assessed in the current study. In addition, one may argue that a second TP is easier to perform due to the anatomic guidance provided by the first TP sheath. Albeit the fact that no direct TP related complications were noted with the participation of a physician-in-training, this excellent outcome may be explained merely by good supervision provided by the staff electrophysiologist.

5 CONCLUSIONS

Transseptal catheterization facilitated by ICE is a feasible and safe alternative to a traditional fluoroscopic approach with a similar rate of complications in patients referred for first-time or redo procedures. This finding appears to be maintained regardless of whether the TP procedure is performed by an experienced invasive electrophysiologist or a physician-in-training under staff supervision. Despite underlying cardiac anatomic abnormalities or increased BMI, it appears that this approach confers a safety profile comparable to centers intimately familiar with the traditional approach to TP. ICE may offer the advantage of direct visualization and optimal positioning of the TP sheath within the LA, as well as providing a wealth of adjunctive imaging data. Importantly, TP facilitates early recognition of potential life-threatening complications. In addition, it may serve best the operator with little experience in TP or centers with low numbers of procedures necessitating a transseptal approach. In order to prove superiority of ICE facilitated over traditional TP, a large-scale prospective head-to-head comparison would be needed in the future.

6 REFERENCES

1. Roelke M, Smith AJ, Palacios IF. The technique and safety of transseptal left heart catheterization: the Massachusetts General Hospital experience with 1,279 procedures. Cathet Cardiovasc Diagn 1994;32:332-9.

2. Cheng A, Calkins H. A conservative approach to performing transseptal punctures without the use of intracardiac echocardiography: stepwise approach with real-time video clips. J Cardiovasc Electrophysiol 2007;18:686-9.

3. De Ponti R, Cappato R, Curnis A, et al. Trans-septal catheterization in the electrophysiology laboratory: data from a multicenter survey spanning 12 years. J Am Coll Cardiol 2006;47:1037-42.

4. Fagundes RL, Mantica M, De Luca L, et al. Safety of single transseptal puncture for ablation of atrial fibrillation: retrospective study from a large cohort of patients. J Cardiovasc Electrophysiol 2007;18:1277-81.

5. Gonzalez MD, Otomo K, Shah N, et al. Transseptal left heart catheterization for cardiac ablation procedures. J Interv Card Electrophysiol 2001;5:89-95.

6. Johnson SB, Seward JB, Packer DL. Phased-array intracardiac echocardiography for guiding transseptal catheter placement: utility and learning curve. Pacing Clin Electrophysiol 2002;25:402-7.

7. Sweeney LJ, Rosenquist GC. The normal anatomy of the atrial septum in the human heart. Am Heart J 1979;98:194-9.

8. Babaliaros V, Block P. State of the art percutaneous intervention for the treatment of valvular heart disease: a review of the current technologies and ongoing research in the field of percutaneous valve replacement and repair. Cardiology 2007;107:87-96.

9. Ross J, Jr., Braunwald E, Morrow AG. Transseptal left atrial puncture; new technique for the measurement of left atrial pressure in man. Am J Cardiol 1959;3:653-5.

10. Brockenbrough EC, Braunwald E, Ross J, Jr. Transseptal left heart catheterization. A review of 450 studies and description of an improved technic. Circulation 1962;25:15-21.

11. Brockenbrough EC, Braunwald E. A new technique for left ventriculography and trans-septal left heart catheterization. Am J Cardiol 1960:1062-1964.

12. Chu E, Fitzpatrick AP, Chin MC, Sudhir K, Yock PG, Lesh MD. Radiofrequency catheter ablation guided by intracardiac echocardiography. Circulation 1994;89:1301-5.

13. Calkins H, Brugada J, Packer DL, et al. HRS/EHRA/ECAS expert consensus statement on catheter and surgical ablation of atrial fibrillation: recommendations for personnel, policy, procedures and follow-up. A report of the Heart Rhythm Society (HRS) Task Force on Catheter and Surgical Ablation of Atrial Fibrillation developed in partnership with the European Heart Rhythm Association (EHRA) and the European Cardiac Arrhythmia Society (ECAS); in collaboration with the American College of Cardiology (ACC), American Heart Association (AHA), and the Society of Thoracic Surgeons (STS). Endorsed and approved by the governing bodies of the American College of Cardiology, the American Heart Association, the European Cardiac Arrhythmia Society, the European Heart Rhythm Association, the Society of Thoracic Surgeons, and the Heart Rhythm Society. Europace 2007;9:335-79.

14. Chu E, Kalman JM, Kwasman MA, et al. Intracardiac echocardiography during radiofrequency catheter ablation of cardiac arrhythmias in humans. J Am Coll Cardiol 1994;24:1351-7.

15. Callans DJ, Wood MA. How to use intracardiac echocardiography for atrial fibrillation ablation procedures. Heart Rhythm 2007;4:242-5.
16. Bruce CJ, Packer DL, Seward JB. Intracardiac Doppler hemodynamics and flow: new vector, phased-array ultrasound-tipped catheter. Am J Cardiol 1999;83:1509-12, A9.
17. Mitchell AR. The emerging role of intracardiac echocardiography – into the ICE age. British Journal of Cardiology 2007;14:31 - 36.
18. Panutich MS, Knight BP. Imaging techniques in cardiac electrophysiology. Expert Rev Cardiovasc Ther 2006;4:59-70.
19. Epstein LM, Mitchell MA, Smith TW, Haines DE. Comparative study of fluoroscopy and intracardiac echocardiographic guidance for the creation of linear atrial lesions. Circulation 1998;98:1796-801.
20. Kalman JM, Fitzpatrick AP, Olgin JE, et al. Biophysical characteristics of radiofrequency lesion formation in vivo: dynamics of catheter tip-tissue contact evaluated by intracardiac echocardiography. Am Heart J 1997;133:8-18.
21. Mangrum JM, Mounsey JP, Kok LC, DiMarco JP, Haines DE. Intracardiac echocardiography-guided, anatomically based radiofrequency ablation of focal atrial fibrillation originating from pulmonary veins. J Am Coll Cardiol 2002;39:1964-72.
22. Marrouche NF, Martin DO, Wazni O, et al. Phased-array intracardiac echocardiography monitoring during pulmonary vein isolation in patients with atrial fibrillation: impact on outcome and complications. Circulation 2003;107:2710-6.
23. Cabrera JA, Sanchez-Quintana D, Ho SY, Medina A, Anderson RH. The architecture of the atrial musculature between the orifice of the inferior caval vein and the tricuspid valve: the anatomy of the isthmus. J Cardiovasc Electrophysiol 1998;9:1186-95.

24. Wood MA, Wittkamp M, Henry D, et al. A comparison of pulmonary vein ostial anatomy by computerized tomography, echocardiography, and venography in patients with atrial fibrillation having radiofrequency catheter ablation. Am J Cardiol 2004;93:49-53.

25. Morton JB, Sanders P, Byrne MJ, et al. Phased-Array intracardiac echocardiography to guide radiofrequency ablation in the left atrium and at the pulmonary vein ostium. J Cardiovasc Electrophysiol 2001;12:343-8.

26. Ren JF, Marchlinski FE, Callans DJ. Left atrial thrombus associated with ablation for atrial fibrillation: identification with intracardiac echocardiography. J Am Coll Cardiol 2004;43:1861-7.

27. Kalman JM, Olgin JE, Karch MR, Hamdan M, Lee RJ, Lesh MD. "Cristal tachycardias": origin of right atrial tachycardias from the crista terminalis identified by intracardiac echocardiography. J Am Coll Cardiol 1998;31:451-9.

28. De Ponti R, Zardini M, Storti C, Longobardi M, Salerno-Uriarte JA. Trans-septal catheterization for radiofrequency catheter ablation of cardiac arrhythmias. Results and safety of a simplified method. Eur Heart J 1998;19:943-50.

29. Hahn K, Gal R, Sarnoski J, Kubota J, Schmidt DH, Bajwa TK. Transesophageal echocardiographically guided atrial transseptal catheterization in patients with normal-sized atria: incidence of complications. Clin Cardiol 1995;18:217-20.

30. Tucker KJ, Curtis AB, Murphy J, et al. Transesophageal echocardiographic guidance of transseptal left heart catheterization during radiofrequency ablation of left-sided accessory pathways in humans. Pacing Clin Electrophysiol 1996;19:272-81.

31. Daoud EG, Kalbfleisch SJ, Hummel JD. Intracardiac echocardiography to guide transseptal left heart catheterization for radiofrequency catheter ablation. J Cardiovasc Electrophysiol 1999;10:358-63.

32. Szili-Torok T, Kimman G, Theuns D, Res J, Roelandt JR, Jordaens LJ. Transseptal left heart catheterisation guided by intracardiac echocardiography. Heart 2001;86:E11.

33. Villacastin J, Castellano NP, Moreno J, Alvarez L, Morales R, Rodriguez A. [Learning process for transseptal puncture guided by intracardiac echocardiography]. Rev Esp Cardiol 2004;57:359-62.

34. Shalganov TN, Paprika D, Borbas S, Temesvari A, Szili-Torok T. Preventing complicated transseptal puncture with intracardiac echocardiography: case report. Cardiovasc Ultrasound 2005;3:5.

35. Shepherd EJ, Gall SA, Furniss SS. Interatrial septal puncture without the use of fluoroscopy-reducing ionizing radiation in left atrial ablation procedures. J Interv Card Electrophysiol 2008;22:183-7.

36. Packer DL, Johnson SB, Kolasa MW, Bunch TJ, Henz BD, Okumura Y. New generation of electro-anatomic mapping: full intracardiac ultrasound image integration. Europace 2008;10 Suppl 3:iii35-41.

37. Tops LF, Schalij MJ, den Uijl DW, Abraham TP, Calkins H, Bax JJ. Image integration in catheter ablation of atrial fibrillation. Europace 2008;10 Suppl 3:iii48-56.

38. Hu YF, Tai CT, Lin YJ, et al. The change in the fluoroscopy-guided transseptal puncture site and difficult punctures in catheter ablation of recurrent atrial fibrillation. Europace 2008;10:276-9.

39. Marcus GM, Ren X, Tseng ZH, et al. Repeat transseptal catheterization after ablation for atrial fibrillation. J Cardiovasc Electrophysiol 2007;18:55-9.

40. Yang HS, Srivathsan K, Wissner E, Chandrasekaran K. Images in cardiovascular medicine. Real-time 3-dimensional transesophageal echocardiography: novel utility in atrial fibrillation ablation with a prosthetic mitral valve. Circulation 2008;117:e304-5.

41. Bidart C, Vaseghi M, Cesario DA, et al. Radiofrequency current delivery via transseptal needle to facilitate septal puncture. Heart Rhythm 2007;4:1573-6.

42. Knecht S, Jais P, Haissaguerre M. Another use for radiofrequency energy during an atrial fibrillation ablation procedure. Europace 2007;9:1142-3.

7 ABREVIATIONS

AO: Aorta

MV: Mitral valve

ICE: Intracardiac echocardiography

EP: Electrophysiology

TP: Transseptal puncture

BMI: Body mass index

AVRT: Atrioventricular reentrant tachycardia

WPW: Wolff-Parkinson-White

AVNRT: Atrioventricular nodal reentrant tachycardia

VT: Ventricular tachycardia

PVC: Premature ventricular contraction

LA: left atrial

AF: Atrial fibrillation

LAVI: Left atrial volume index

TEE: Transesophageal echocardiography

LVEF: Left ventricular ejection fraction

D: Double

S: Single

SVC: Superior vena cava

RA: Right atrium

RIPV: Right inferior pulmonary vein

RSPV: Right superior pulmonary vein

LIPV: Left inferior pulmonary vein

LSPV: Left superior pulmonary vein

TV: Tricuspid valve

8 Figures and Tables

Figure 1. Interatrial septum and limbus encircling the fossa ovalis seen from a right atrial view (from (8))

Figure 2. Original setup used in Dr. Brockenbrough's study describing transseptal catheterization in 450 patients. Needle 'C' shows the Brockenbrough needle used today.

Table 1. Comparison between Mechanical (Rotational) and Phased-Array ICE (adapted from (15,18))

Figure 3. The "home" view displays right atrium, right ventricle and tricuspid valve. *RA*, right atrium; *TV*, tricuspid valve; *RV*, right ventricle. Image courtesy of Siemens Corporation

Figure 4. View of intra-atrial septum and fossa ovalis. *RA*, right atrium; *LA*, left atrium. Image courtesy of Siemens Corporation

Figure 5. View of superior and inferior left pulmonary veins. *RA*, right atrium; *LA*, left atrium; *LSPV*, left superior pulmonary vein; *LIPV*, left inferior pulmonary vein. Image courtesy of Siemens Corporation

Figure 6. View of right superior and inferior pulmonary veins. *SVC*, superior vena cava; *RSPV*, right superior pulmonary vein; *RIPV*, right inferior pulmonary vein. Image courtesy of Siemens Corporation

Figure 7. Left ventricle in long axis view for the assessment of pericardial effusion. *LV*, left ventricle; *LA*, left atrium; *AO*, aorta; *MV*, mitral valve. Image courtesy of Siemens Corporation

Figure 8. Intracardiac echocardiography image demonstrating a lipomatous septum with transseptal catheter traversing a narrow fossa ovalis

Table 2. Clinical Application of Intracardiac Echocardiography

Table 3. Baseline Demographic & Echocardiographic Data of the Patients, N=167 (%)

Table 4. Type of Procedure Among the Cohort of Patients (N=167)

Table 5. Number of Patients with Redo Procedures

Table 6. Transseptal Punctures

Table 7. Intraprocedural Complications Among the Patient Cohort (N=167)

Table 8. Pericardial Effusions Noted During Next Day Limited Echocardiographic Evaluation in 118 Patients

Table 9. Pericardial Effusions Noted During Next Day Limited Echocardiographic Evaluation in 20 Redo Patients

Table 10. Echocardiographic Parameters

Figure 9. Right atrial NavX map with tenting of the needle tip visualized along the fossa ovalis (white arrow head; yellow dots mark the His bundle position). From (35)

Figure 10. CartoSound image of the left atrium realized through integration of ICE imaging and electroanatomic mapping. In addition, CT image integration visualizing the pulmonary veins is shown. From (37)

Figure 11A. Tenting of the fossa ovalis (black arrow head) by the transseptal catheter tip (white arrow head) as seen from the left atrial perspective. From (40)

Figure 11B. The ablation catheter is visualized traversing the intra-atrial septum from right to left atrium following successful transseptal puncture. From (40)

9   DANKSAGUNG

Mein Dank gilt Prof. Dr. med Karl-Heinz Kuck und Dr. med. Julian Chun zum Anstoß und der Betreuung dieser Arbeit. Zudem bedanke ich mich bei meinem Mentor und Freund Gregory T. Altemose, MD. Mein Dank gilt auch meiner Frau Halla und meinem Sohn Noah, ohne deren Geduld diese Doktorarbeit nicht hätte entstehen können. Vor allem möchte ich mich bei meinen Eltern, Hannah Wißner-Heesch, Michael Heesch, Inge Wißner und Erich Wißner bedanken, die mich bei all meinen Vorhaben stets unterstützt haben.

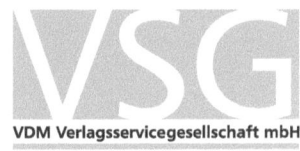

Die VDM Verlagsservicegesellschaft sucht für wissenschaftliche Verlage abgeschlossene und herausragende

Dissertationen, Habilitationen, Diplomarbeiten, Master Theses, Magisterarbeiten usw.

für die kostenlose Publikation als Fachbuch.

Sie verfügen über eine Arbeit, die hohen inhaltlichen und formalen Ansprüchen genügt, und haben Interesse an einer honorarvergüteten Publikation?

Dann senden Sie bitte erste Informationen über sich und Ihre Arbeit per Email an *info@vdm-vsg.de*.

Sie erhalten kurzfristig unser Feedback!

VDM Verlagsservicegesellschaft mbH
Dudweiler Landstr. 99   Telefon +49 681 3720 174
D - 66123 Saarbrücken   Fax   +49 681 3720 1749
www.vdm-vsg.de

Die VDM Verlagsservicegesellschaft mbH vertritt

 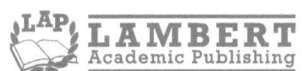 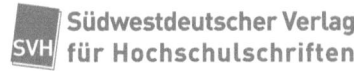

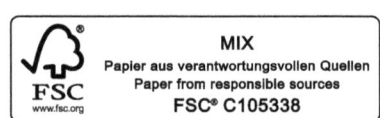

Printed by Books on Demand GmbH, Norderstedt / Germany